REAL SECRETS
OF YOUNG AND FRESH LOOKING
SKIN
FROM FRENCH BEAUTIES

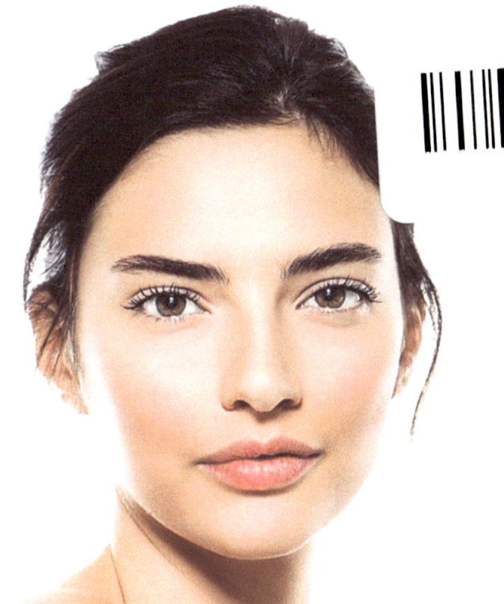

+HOMEMADE LIFTING MASKS RECIPES
+PEELING RECIPES
+FRESH SKIN MASKS

SOFI BELL

"There Is Nothing Mysterious or Difficult

About Giving Yourself

the Most Beautiful Face in the World"

Estee Lauder

Table of Contents

How Do French Women Manage to Look Younger than Women from Other Countries?

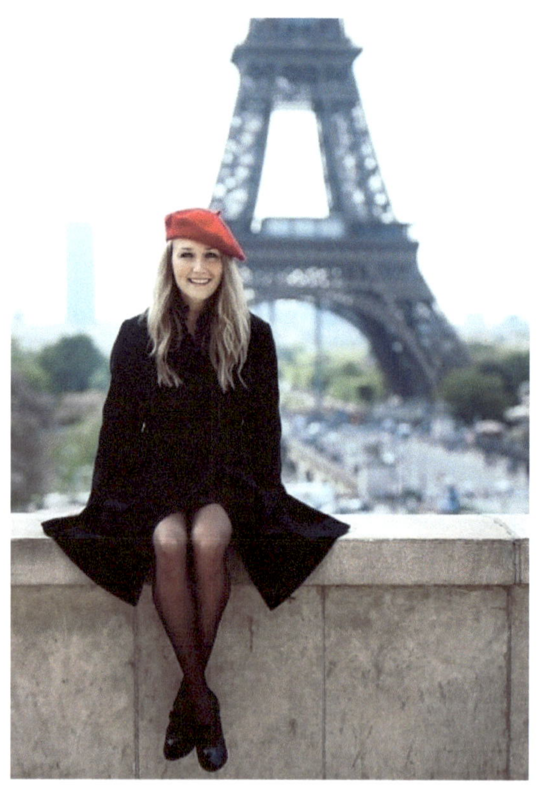

French women tend to age slowly when compared to women from other countries. Did you ever wonder how this is possible?

It is never an easy task to guess the age of a French actress. For example, if you look at Cotillard, you will think that she is only around 30-35 years old. But in reality, she is 41 years old. She is a perfect example to prove that French women age slowly when compared to others. In general, a French woman is around 1.5 times younger when compared to a British woman. This has left a question on the minds of most people who live out there in the world.

The answer to this question is a simple one. All the women in France start to look after their skin at a younger age. Then they follow some skincare treatments on a regular basis, along with the assistance of some high-quality products. This help them to eliminate the adverse effects of aging conveniently. This can be provided with statistical figures as well, and it has been discovered that women who live in France spend around £1.9 annually to purchase anti-aging products. This annual figure supersedes the total spent by women in Spain, Germany, and the UK put together and could be the reason why they have such glowing skin, not only limited to their faces but all over their bodies as well.

This is a clear example available to prove how much French women are concerned about the skin.

French women do not just spend their money to purchase skincare and anti-aging products; they also prefer to spend a considerable amount of time on a daily basis to take care of the skin. In fact, French women spend twice the time that British women spend when taking care of the skin.

French women don't follow any magical methods to reverse the adverse effects associated with aging, they just use few simple techniques to make sure that they look good at all times. Hence, any person can also follow these techniques to ensure the good looks.

If you want to make your skin look like that of a French woman, you will need to cleanse your skin, tone it, and moisturize on a regular basis. It is better if you can get the assistance of a high-quality serum. It can contribute towards the results that you will get at the end of the day. However, you need to make sure that you don't use multiple products to make your skin look good. If you use multiple products, there is a higher possibility for you to end up with negative results.

It is a good idea to invest money in some high-quality serums, it can be considered as one of the secrets on how French women tend to maintain great looking skins. The best quality skin serums come along with highly efficient formulas; they go deep into your skin and eliminate all the negative signs of aging, including wrinkles and fine lines. French women never forget the importance of a décolletage. Most of the women tend to apply the serums and creams only down to the jawline, but French women prefer to apply the serums and creams on their chests as well. As a result, they maintain the great looks of the entire body.

French women also tend to incorporate massages into their regular skincare regime. In other words, they have a clear understanding of the importance of facial massages, with the help of circular massaging movements; they boost the circulation of blood in the face, this provided them with a healthy flushed glow as well. In addition, these massaging techniques plump and firm the skin along with time. Hence, all women can think about incorporating it into the regular skincare regime.

Also, you need to keep in mind that French women don't just rely on foundation, this is a common mistake done by women who live in other parts of the world; they are looking forward to investing heavily on foundations. As a result, they are incapable of getting rid of all the imperfections in the skin, including eliminating wrinkles and fine lines on the skin.

Famous beauties of France

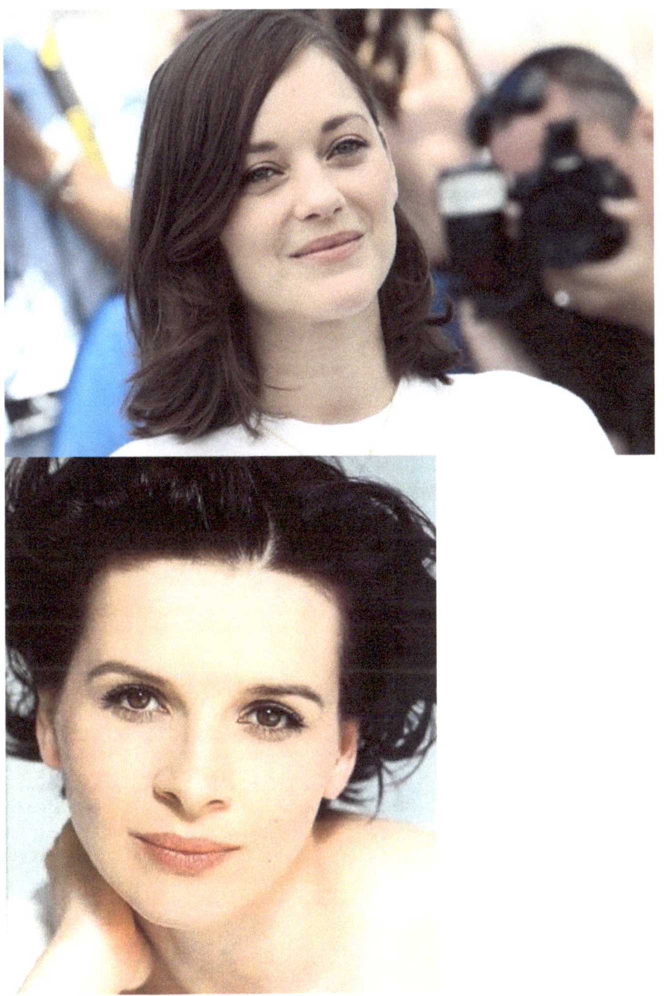

Marion Cotoll and Juliett Binoche

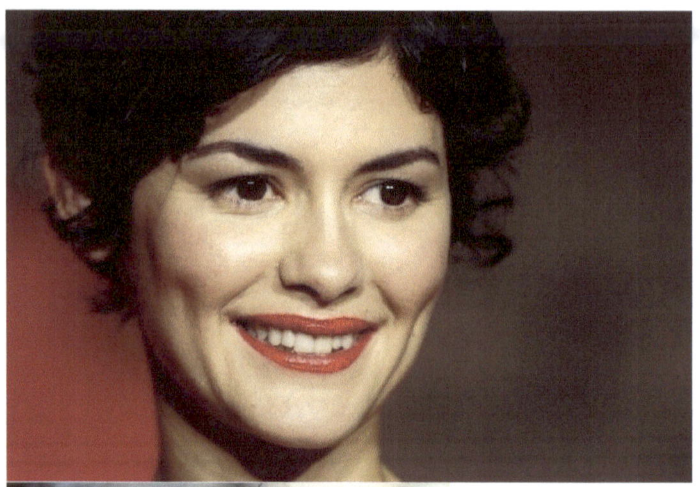

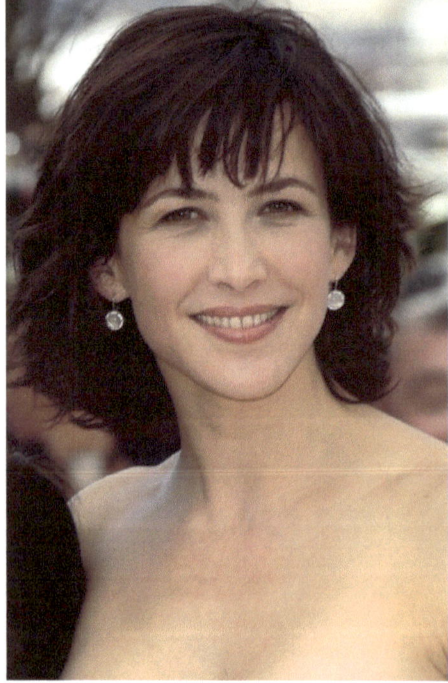

Audrey Tautoe and Sophie Marceau

What Are the Main Reasons for Skin Aging?

The structure and use of our skin

The internal organs, ligaments, bones, muscles, nerves, and blood vessels are all held in place by the covering that our body is wrapped with, all over us, which is the skin.

When the skin is damaged, we bleed, and that is because it is full of blood vessels, and when these are cut or split open the blood flows out.

This wrap around, that we call the skin is about 1.5 to 2.0 square meters (16.10 to 21.50 square feet), in an average man and without we would look horrible and vulnerable to disease and sickness.

The skin protects us from the elements, harsh environmental conditions, weather and climatic changes, the sun, dusts, etc. And ensures that we are well protected, in turn, it is our duty to reciprocate the care and look after our skin, so that it is cared for adequately and especially that our skin is not damaged from anything that is around us.

Many things in Nature could damage our skin, the Sun, the wind, the air, water, fire and the list just goes on.

Reasons behind skin aging

Here is a list of some of the most prominent factors that can lead towards skin aging.

1. Sun – Sun can be considered as one of the biggest culprits behind skin aging. If you are constantly exposed to the sun for a long period, there is a higher possibility that your skin will end up with a Sun massive damage.
2. Smoking – From the recent studies, it has been discovered that people who smoke are more vulnerable towards skin damages when compared to others.

3. Low carb and protein intake – If your carb intake and the protein intake are low, you will experience a higher degree of skin aging, they are two of the essential nutrients that you should take in to maintain your external appearance.

4. Not consuming enough vegetables and fruits – You are strongly encouraged to include a lot of fresh vegetables and fruits in your meals. Failing to do it can faster the rate of skin aging. However, if you consume fresh fruits and vegetables, your body will get the ability to eliminate toxins and help you retain skin health.

5. Generics – Generics has also been identified as one of the main reasons that lead people towards the signs of aging.

6. Lack of sleep – If you don't take enough sleep, you will have to deal with the negative consequences associated with damaged skin.

7. Alcohol – Just like smoking, the consumption of alcohol has been one of the agents that can lead you towards premature aging.

Good skin care

It is imperative that we take a good care of our skin, as it is our first line of defense and with age our skin ages. If we could care for it we could help to delay the process, and that is what many of us would want because if we could have a radiant skin, we would look younger than our age.

There are many ways that we could care for our skin and the best we could do is to nourish it from the inside, we try to do so from the outside.

To nourish our skin from the inside, we would need to ensure that we consume a balanced diet, which would help our body and our organs to feed nourishments through our blood vessels to the skin.

We need to feed the skin with some vital vitamins for its maintenance and continuous growth and wellbeing. And some of them which would help are vitamins, A, D, C and E. Along with supplementing these vital nutrients we would also need to eat fruits, vegetables, fibrous food and drink a lot of water to ensure that our skin is kept well hydrated.

While we ensure a good supply of what the skin needs from the inside, it would also be prudent to care for it from the outside too, and for such an endeavor, there are many ways in which we could accomplish that.

With the advent of various creams and other skin care products that are prolifically sold around the world and are available to us, we need to very carefully in selecting what we would apply on our skin, especially the face, which is the most sensitive part of the skin, and if we are careless, we could end up with much more than what we bargained for in the end.

The most prudent way of using any creams for the first time even if you have been using the product for years would be to first apply a little of the cream on the underside of your upper arm, under the armpit and keep it for a couple of hours. And then, if there is no adverse effect, you can apply on the face.

This is because even if there are no changes in the composition of the cream since you last used it, that particular pack could have had a problem in manufacture or your skin could have undergone some changes and by doing so, if there is any adverse reaction you could easily treat it, unlike if it was on your face.

- ***Skin Cleansing***

Cleaning your skin especially the facial tissues is very important if you want to retain the gloss in your skin and by cleaning it regularly, you could remove all the dirt and grime that would embed into it when you are exposed.

- ***Exfoliation***

Our skin continually sheds itself, and new skin is formed which is a continuously occurring phenomenon, and some of these "dead skin" particles could remain on our faces, and by cleaning it, which is popularly called a facial, we could remove it and ensure the healthier skin is exposed.

- ***Humidification***

Your skin needs to retain the water it holds within at all times but when it is cold or even hot weather, the outsider skin could lose water hence you would need to use a humidifier.

Either it could be in the form of a cream or hot steam to open up the pores and ensure that the skin is allowed to breathe and take in water that is in the atmosphere, to keep the skin moist.

- ***Protection***

The skin protects us, and we need to protect our skin, and the best way to do so would be to ensure that we take in ample amount of water and eat nourishing food, which would be the best we could do for the wellbeing of our skin.

We are vulnerable to the Ultra Violet rays of the Sun, which could be harmful to our skin especially when we are exposed to it for a very long time.

Those of us who would go to the beach or indulge in various outdoor sports are exposed to the Sun for long hours; we should protect ourselves with a good quality "sunscreen" which would effectively keep the harmful rays of the Sun away.

Skin cancers are formed when we are exposed to long hours out in the Sun. Hence, special care is imperative.

How French Women Take Care of Their Skin All Through Their Lives

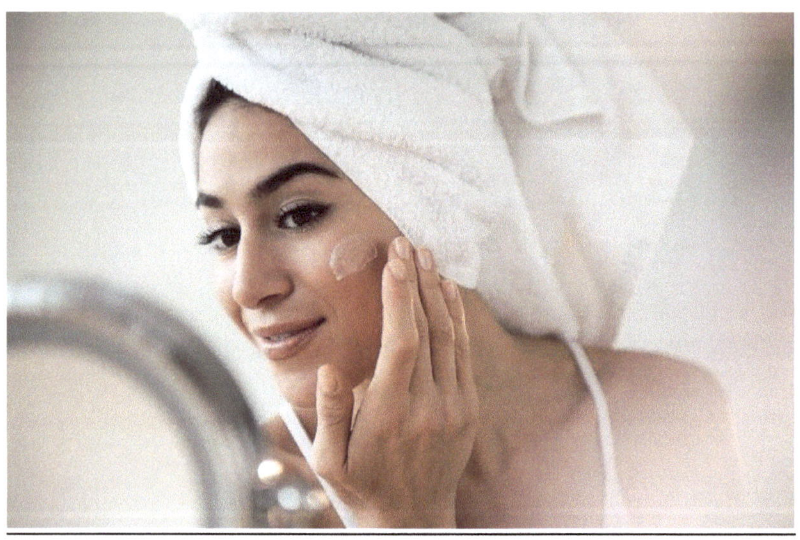

The big divide

Paris and New York are both fashion capitals of the world, but they are divided by a gigantic body of water, the Atlantic Ocean, which could be the secret to women in France aging gracefully while their counterparts on the wrong side of the Atlantic do not.

Is it the breeze from the West to the East across the Atlantic, which soothes the skin of the women in France and leaves them as young as ever all through their lives or is there a bigger secret, which is kept secretly hidden within the confines of every French home?

This annual figure supersedes the total spent by women in Spain, Germany, and the UK put together and could be the reason that they have such glowing skin, not only limited to their faces but all over their bodies as well.

If you happen to use the bathroom in a French home, it would be filled with an assortment of many types of cosmetics used all over the body and would look like a cosmetic kiosk, round the corner, down the street.

Whether this is the secret to their ever-glowing skin, we would not know, but apart from that, French women have something about them, which keeps them at heart, as well as in looks for most of their lives.

Starting young

They do start early, and it would not be surprising to see French girls as young as 13 or around 15, who would be quite conscious of the fact that looking as beautiful as they could is a national trait more than anything else is.

It is an inborn instinct that radiates around the fairer sex among the French, and they do facilitate the requirements to being young by helping themselves to put the brakes on premature aging unlike those women across the Atlantic.

They would always remain conscious that keeping the weight down is much easier than putting it down and it is not that they do not feed themselves adequately, as France is known to be a gastronomic cauldron of international gourmet.

Skin care massage.

French women like to do facials professionally, or home massages because they like what their reflection looks like in the mirror after this procedure. Massage saturates the skin with oxygen and strengthens it. For the skin, it is the same training as for your session in the gym, and it should be consistent. Often working people in France do not have the opportunity to get a professional massage because they would rather spend free time with the family.

However, they do not forget about the daily facial massage. French women can quickly do this procedure at home in front of the TV, in the company of children and her husband. For the French massage procedure, choose facial and oil creams with lightweight, non-greasy, non-tacky textures.

By the way, the process of massage helps useful components from the means to penetrate into the thick layers of the skin and actively work for the benefit of its healing and rejuvenation. As for the massage technique, each woman chooses them herself, depending on the needs of the skin.

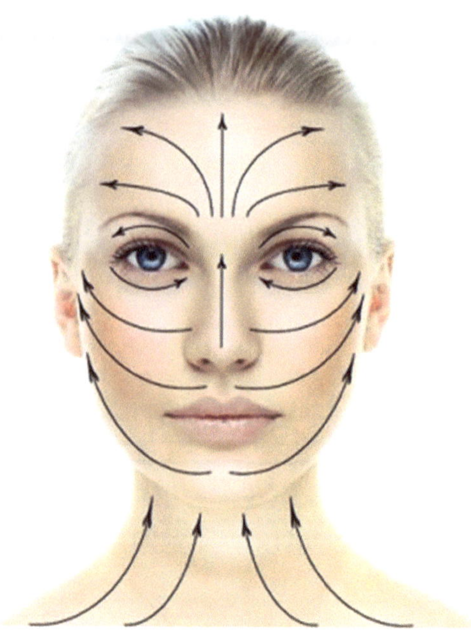

Facial massage lines, eyelids and décolleté

Eating healthy

France has a broader variety of food to choose from than any other country in mainland Europe, as it is the gateway to the Mediterranean and the delights of the Middle East, and of the African continent.

If we have our doubts that the French women do not enjoy their food, we may have to think again as they are excellent cooks too compared to those across the Atlantic, and this has been written through the ages and it is never in dispute.

The secret to maintaining their figures would mostly depend on the way they consume their food, rather than eating significant portions like most women across the Atlantic, they eat just morsels at a time and would do it more often rather than at traditional times.

They habitually step onto the weighing scale in the bathroom to check on their progress in keeping the weight down, and as soon as the scale tips to the right, they would ensure that it is brought back to where it was.

It is their overall health consciousness that keeps their skin glowing as they gracefully age and with the weight down to manageable proportions it would reflect on their overall body structure, skin, and general health.

Pampering oneself

French women have an inherent habit of spoiling themselves and they would indulge in specific natural skin uplifting technique that has been tried and tested. Like for instance the "Thalassotherapy."

Thalassotherapy is a seawater-based treatment that originated from France, which uses water jets, seaweed wraps, mud baths, and sea fog inhalation.

This therapy is known to improve blood circulation, promote better sleeping, tone the muscles, and reduce the incidence of cellulite in the body.

They would also spend hours if given the opportunity of time to soak themselves in a luxuriating bath filled with a variety of perfumed and specially selected soaps to ensure that they keep the skin as clean and nourished as possible.

Projecting confidence

French women also exude tons of confidence, which helps them to keep their facial muscles in the right shape, and could be another reason why they bring out the best in them even when stepping out to walk down to the grocery.

France is known for its fashion and turning out best is what most French women practice as a habit. It may be elegant and eye-catching which is not limited only to its capital but it is a part of their lifestyle.

Cosmetic surgery is not popular in France though some women may try it out in extreme cases, overall they tend to maintain their profiles as best as they could to look as natural as they could be.

It is also a prevalent notion among the elder women passing their prime to inculcate in their young charges that there is a certain age for women to look beautiful to be loved and likewise there is an age where they need to be loved to look beautiful.

Walking the best exercise

Gyms are not so popular in France, and they have the notion that they could walk just anywhere and get themselves into shape, instead of needing a treadmill.

This way, we would see so many women in Paris, the suburbs and even in the countryside enjoying their walks and taking long walks, which are a habit that is inculcated in them since they were young.

Lastly, it is a perennial notion that French women are good lovers, are good in bed, have a healthy body, a healthy mind, good and happy sex may be an essential criterion.

Therefore, when all the good things add up in life, it is not only the skin that would glow, the women in France would too, and that is what we see around us when we step out onto the street.

Face Lifting Care

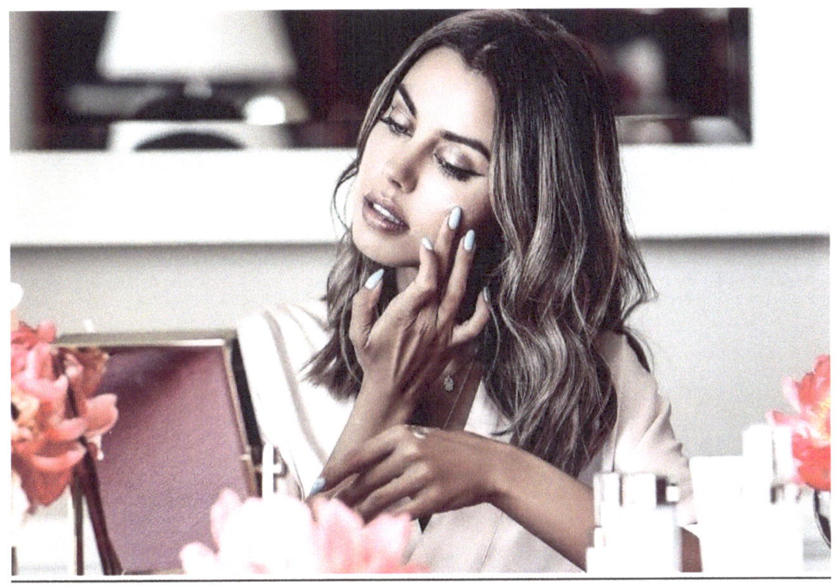

Our skin is the first line of defense that we have against all the climatic conditions we are exposed to especially in our environment. The skin ages as we age. All ethnicities would show aging of the skin without any exception, but by proper skin care, the process of aging could be slowed down by keeping the skin well nourished and protecting it especially from the Sun.

Aging of the skin is also seen when the process where dead skin, which is supposed to shed off regularly from our body and the new skin that grows underneath to take over, is slowed down and with regular exfoliation, this could be corrected.

Exfoliation which is the removal of dead skin needs to be regular with the aging process expediting the new skin to take over and if we do not do so, the aging of the skin would not only be seen it would also occur faster.

When we care for our face, which is the most sensitive part of our skin, and undergo what we refer to as "facials" it is indeed the process of shedding that we employ to remove the old skin and bring the new skin out and keep it nourished and glowed.

The process of shedding also helps to retain water in the skin and to smooth out the lines especially on the face and restore the Sun damaged skin back to what it was, but this does not mean that the aging process would stop, it would only help to slow down.

Types of Face Lifting Care and procedures

There are many ways that you could employ face lifting, and the most practiced is by consuming a properly balanced diet to ensure that all the vitamins required for good healthy skin are naturally supplied from within our system.

- Some of the essential vitamins that the face would need to be well nourished from within would be, A, D, C and E among many others and ensuring that these ate taken into your system in the appropriate quantities regularly would help.

- The other procedure that we could employ would be the use of proper external care for the skin, and these would be natural applications, which would not have any allergic reactions on the skin, especially the face.

- The third would be to use reputed brands of cosmetics, which would revitalize and rejuvenate the skin and ensure that the aging process is slowed down giving the skin a more healthy and glowing look even if aging catches up on you which is of course, inevitable.

- The other would be to conduct plastic surgery for skin lifting which could be an expensive and painful procedure and could even have after effects, which you would have to contend with.

Of the above the priority would be to enhance the skin and the care for it by a balanced diet, of with natural external procedures, cosmetics could also help and if no allergies are detected could be acceptable, but surgery should be avoided at all costs because they are dangerous procedures still.

Do it at home

- *How often*

It is necessary to know your type of skin before you attempt to do any skin care at home, as there are different types of skin, which would need applications.

There is sensitive, healthy, oily, dry and combination skin, hence identifying the type you have would be desirable before you employ any method of exfoliation on your face.

The two types of procedures that you can employ; one is mechanical and the other chemical.

Your kind of skin should to guide the kind that you would choose.

Mechanical procedures involve using a brush, scrub, or sponge that would physically remove dead skin from the body and in the chemical process; you could use mild Alpha and Beta hydroxyl acids to dissolve dead skin gently.

The regularity of conducting exfoliation on your skin would depend on the type of skin you have and the type of method that you choose, but it is necessary that you do not overdo it, hence consulting an approved dermatologist would be in your better interests.

- *The order to follow*

It is essential that you follow a proper sequence when conducting face lifting care or exfoliation and the best procedure would be to remove all dead skin from the body especially on the face by either mechanical or chemical method while care is to be taking not to damage your skin.

Then an appropriate facemask, which would suit your type of skin, could be applied on, and after its removal, a gentle massage would revitalize and rejuvenate your skin.

Homemade Peeling Recipes

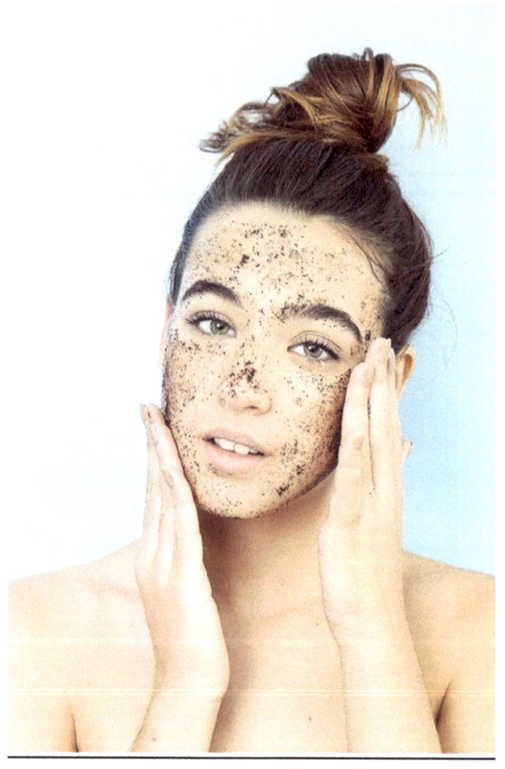

Peeling is a procedure aimed at cleansing the skin by exfoliating the keratinized cells. Conducted according to all the rules, manipulation allows you to get rid of fine wrinkles, fresh pimples, and traces from them, improve the color and texture of the facial skin, narrow the pores, and get rid of many common problems.

The cleansing procedure removes the dead cells from the skin. In cosmetic practice, mechanical, laser, chemical varieties are used that have a superficial, medium, or profound effect on the face. As a rule, at home, use mechanical peeling. It affects the upper or middle layers of the epidermis, removes dead cells from the skin, improves complexion, stimulates the regeneration of the skin, tightens, and tones.

To cope with age-related changes, deep peeling is required. It is carried out by the action of chemicals (acid), specialized equipment (laser), therefore this kind of purification procedure, as a rule, is performed in cosmetic hospitals. The use of mechanical peeling (scrub) of the face at home is based on the addition of various abrasive substances (crushed nuts, salt, cereals, etc.) in cosmetics.

Solid particles scrape the cornified scales from the skin and massage its surface. In case of a normal, healthy skin, it is enough to apply a scrub once a week. For oily skin, more resistant to mechanical effects, the peeling procedure is performed after 3 days. Dry skin requires gentle care, so the scrub is applied once every 10 days. Peeling is prohibited if the face has cracks or inflammation

For superficial peeling, special preparation is not needed. It is enough just to make make-up and remove sebum and dirt with a natural lotion or tonic, apply peeling remedy and after a while to wash off.

Using natural ingredients found commonly, you could prepare a face-peeling mask that would not be harmful or have any adverse effects like for instance when you use chemical based cosmetic preparations.

• *Wrinkle-free facial peel*

½ cup of seedless cucumber pulp

One white of egg

I tablespoon of strained lemon juice

Mix all the ingredients well and apply gently on the face with a brush, leave to dry thoroughly and after slowly peel it off and leave the face without rinsing for about another half hour. Then rinse with lukewarm water and dry with a soft towel.

• *Dead skin removing facial peel*

½ cup of pulp of fresh pineapple

¼ cup of pulp of fresh papaya

½ tablespoon of bee honey

Mix all the ingredients well into a paste and gently apply on the face and the entire neck with a brush, using fingers could transfer bacteria from fingers to face. Leave for about half an hour until the paste dries up well, then gently remove, rinse with lukewarm water, and dry with a soft towel.

• *pH restoration facial peel*

Pulp from one fresh ripe tomato

1 packet gelatin unflavored

2 tablespoons full, fresh orange juice

Heat up the gelatin and once dissolved add the pulp of tomato.

Add the orange juice when it is cooled and mix them up well.

After cooling, apply to face and neck and leave for 20 minutes to completely dry.

Remove and then leave for another 10 minutes.

Rinse with lukewarm water and dry with a soft towel

• *Facial peel for skin glow*

One yolk of egg

I tablespoon full of bee honey

¼ cup of lime juice

One packet of unflavored gelatin

Mix all the ingredients into a paste. Apply gently on the face and neck. Leave the paste on for about 30 minutes until well dried. Then peel off gently.

Rinse with lukewarm water and dry with a soft towel

• *Peeling for the fading skin of the face*

Blend in a coffee grinder dried lemon zest, 1 tsp. Zest mix with 1 tsp. Oat flakes, add 1 Tsp our cream or vegetable oil, egg yolk.

Egg yolk carefully grinds with sour cream, add flakes, zest, sour cream, or butter, mix thoroughly.

Apply the composition to the skin of the face, rubbing it on the massage lines; leave the layer for 20 minutes. Afterwards, wash off the mask with a warm, then with cold water.

Therefore, there are ample fresh fruits, vegetables, and other ingredients, freely available to us at minimal cost, which we can use without any fear of adverse reactions or allergies.

Using these in a combination would provide us enough natural vitamins and other values, bringing out the best in our skin, and the added bonus is that they are very efficient compared to visiting a beautician to get a facial peel done, especially with a load of chemicals on our face.

Homemade Lifting Masks Recipes for Face

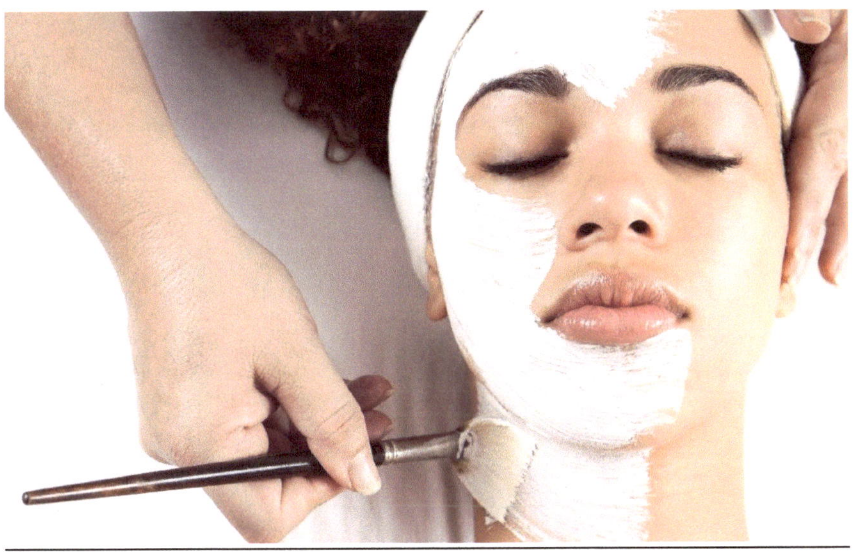

Ensuring that we maintain a proper healthy diet is supplying all the vitamins needed to keep our skin well-nourished and in the meantime also looking after it by using the proper skin creams, sunscreens, and moisturizers we could keep our skin as healthy as it should be.

We could nourish our skin from the inside as well as from the outside, and this dual strategy could be adopted to ensure we have a good skin, which would look healthy and be healthy at any time of the day.

Face masks, which are essential to exfoliate our facial skin, if carried out regularly would remove all dead skin on the face, revitalize, and rejuvenate the look.

Wearing face masks at home would require of us some level of understanding, as it has to be adequately prepared and with the right ingredients or it could do more harm than good for some of us.

Below is the list of the best five but simple to prepare face mask recipes, using natural ingredients which you can prepare at home without much ado:

The Recipes

- Wash clean and cut a few fresh cabbage leaves.

Blend or chop into a paste

Add bee honey and yogurt

If you have a dry skin- add a teaspoon of almond oil

Apply this mask all over the face, neck, and Collette with a brush and leave it to dry for about 15 minutes, and then rinse with lukewarm water and dry with a soft towel.

- Wash peel and cut a fresh chilled cucumber

Blend it into a paste

Add an egg white and a teaspoon of lemon juice

Add a few drops of vitamin E oil

Mix everything well

Apply all over the face, neck, and Collette with a brush, leave for about 20 minutes and once dry rinse with lukewarm water and pat dry with soft towel.

- Small cup of heavy whipping cream

One ripe banana mashed in the cream

Add contents of a vitamin E capsule

Mix well

Apply on face, neck, and Collette with a brush and lie flat on your back for 15 minutes.

Gently wipe off the dried mask with a soft wet cloth and then rinse with lukewarm water.

- Blend or mix well the pulp of Avocado, bee honey, and egg white

Apply gently with a brush on the face, neck, and Collette.

Leave to dry for about 20 minutes by lying on your back.

Rinse with lukewarm water and dry with soft cloth.

- Mix one white of egg with vitamin "E" from two capsules and mix well

Then add one teaspoon of lemon juice.

Make it into a paste and leave it in the refrigerator for half an hour.

Apply evenly with a brush on the face, neck, and Collette.

Leave mask to dry up, around 20 minutes completely.

Then rinse with lukewarm water and dry with soft towel.

Techniques to apply correctly

- ***Face***

Wash face well with a good face wash.

Scrub the face if using a face mask but only once a week.

Wash again and rinse with lukewarm water.

Apply face mask evenly with a brush and not with a brush.

The brush should move from bottom to top, on the face, then neck and then the Collette.

Never apply facemask from top to bottom.

When rinsing to remove the facemask, ensure that you do it from bottom to top too.

- ***Under eyes***

The facemask should be applied with a brush specially kept clean to use whenever you would want to.

Move brush from one side only, from inside the face under the eyes to the outside towards the ear.

The movement should be slow and gentle.

Apply well to eyes while the eye is kept closed.

The same procedure should be practiced if you are applying the facemask on your decollete as well and leaving it for the same period and then rinsing it well and drying with a towel.

If you regularly wear clothes that would expose your shoulders and are out in the Sun for long, it would be advisable that you apply a facemask on your decollete to ensure that you keep it well-nourished and exfoliated.

Applying sunscreen when you are out would also be important as your skin could suffer damage, and being in the Sun regularly could have detrimental effects and even cause skin cancer.

Homemade Facial Mask Recipe for a Fresh Skin

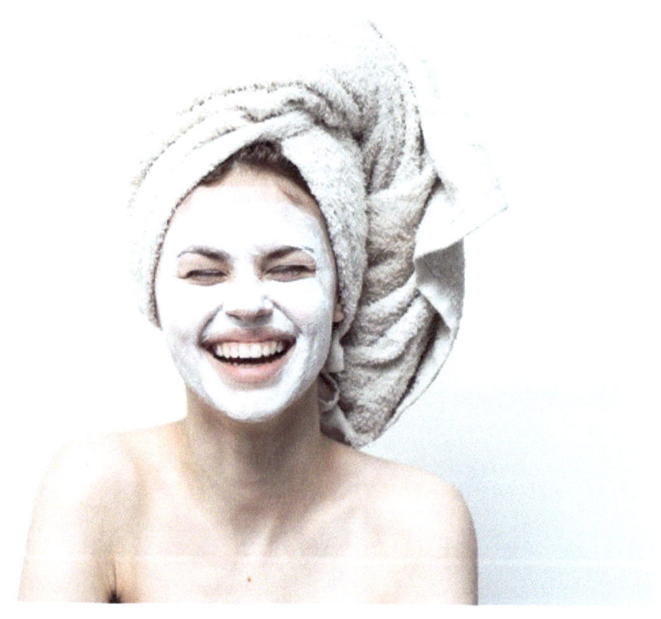

The amount of money you spend to keep yourself looking naturally can be overwhelming, with the ever-increasing cost of getting facial masks and removing dirt and impurities from your skin, one will ask whether or not there exist an homemade DIY recipes and masks that could help reduce or eliminate the experience of acquiring a facial mask. Here are (9) homemade facial mask recipes that are as effective as the ones you will get anywhere.

- ***Banana facial mask***

With banana, you would not have to pay so high to get Botox. Banana offers a tremendously inexpensive alternative for moisturizing the skin. It can be used as an all-natural homemade facial mask for making the skin feel softer and look tender. This highly efficient facial cream is made by mashing up a ripe banana into a somewhat paste. This cream (paste) can then be applied to the face and neck and allowed on the face for about 10 to 20 minutes after which it can then be rinsed. A combination of banana, yogurt, and honey also produces what is regarded by many as the best homemade face mask.

- ## *Yogurt facial mask*

Looking for a quick, easy, and effective way of cleaning and tightening up pores in your skin? Yogurt homemade mask offers your face the quick face assist it needs, and just like many other homemade facial masks, all it will take is between 10 to 20 minutes for it to work its magic. To make this face mask, all you need do is to mix a tablespoon of yogurt (plain yogurt), a quarter of an orange, a few of the orange pulp, a teaspoon of Aloe Vera. In less than five minutes after the application of this mixture, you will begin to feel it working

- ## *Egg facial mask*

If you have a dry skin and you are looking for something to help keep your skin moisturized, then, an egg facial mask may be all that you need. Don't have dry skin and you are wondering whether or not this mask recipe is for you too, well, yes. All can use this mask recipe; the only thing that should be noted is that the skin type determines how it will be used. For someone with dry skin, you will have to separate the egg and then beat the yolk, for someone with an oily skin, remove the yolk; all you need is the white. For someone with normal skin, you need the whole egg. Irrespective of the skin type, correctly use the egg face mask. After half an hour, you will love our new face.

- ***Vinegar facial mask***

It has been known for age long that vinegar is as effective in toning, as it is in ripping the skin clear of dirt. This is one of the most comfortable homemade face masks there is, all you need is a quarter of a cup of vinegar and the same quantity of water. Applying this solution guarantees an effective cleaning and the feeling of confidence that comes with it.

- ***Milk facial mask***

Milk is another recipe for a fantastic facial spar. It provides another way to beautify your face. It can be made by mixing powdered milk with water in such a way that the milk is as thick as a paste. It is this paste that you will apply to your face. After 20 to 30 minutes, you can then wash it off. Having done this, you are left with a rejuvenated skin that is fresh and exquisite.

- ***Oatmeal facial masks***

Oatmeal is your go facial mask if you are looking for something quick to leave you looking and feeling fantastic. Half a cup of hot water, a third of a cup of oatmeal, two spoons of sugar, plain yogurt, two spoons of honey and an egg white is all you need. After it has been mixed, it can be applied to your face and left for 10 to 20, minutes. After rinsing it, you are left with a fantastic look.

- ***Mustard facial mask***

This is another interesting and more or less, free homemade facial rejuvenation way. It braces your face and stimulates the skin to make a beautiful look.

- ***Mayonnaise Facial masks***

What is the point of wasting your money buying expensive facial creams to make masks when you can make yourself a homemade face mask out of an egg mayonnaise? This mayonnaise can be spread gently on your face and left for 10 to 20 minutes after which it can now be washed off.

- ***Honey facial mask***

Honey is a very popular anti-bacterial, it is also well known for its incredible ability to heal and rejuvenate, and this is what makes it such an excellent facial mask recipe. This nourishing facial mask can be made by brewing a cup of chamomile tea with raw honey and a spoon of yeast. When mixing, enough chamomile tea should be taken; and excess should be guided against to ensure that the solution is still thick enough to be applied to the face, 15 to 20 minutes after it has been applied, it can be rinsed out

As our skin types are different so are the creams best for our skins, for sure, we cannot categorically highlight the best of them all, but careful use of them will unravel the most efficient for your skin that you may regard as your best facial mask.

The Ultimate Tips for Living, Staying Pretty and Young as Revealed by French Women

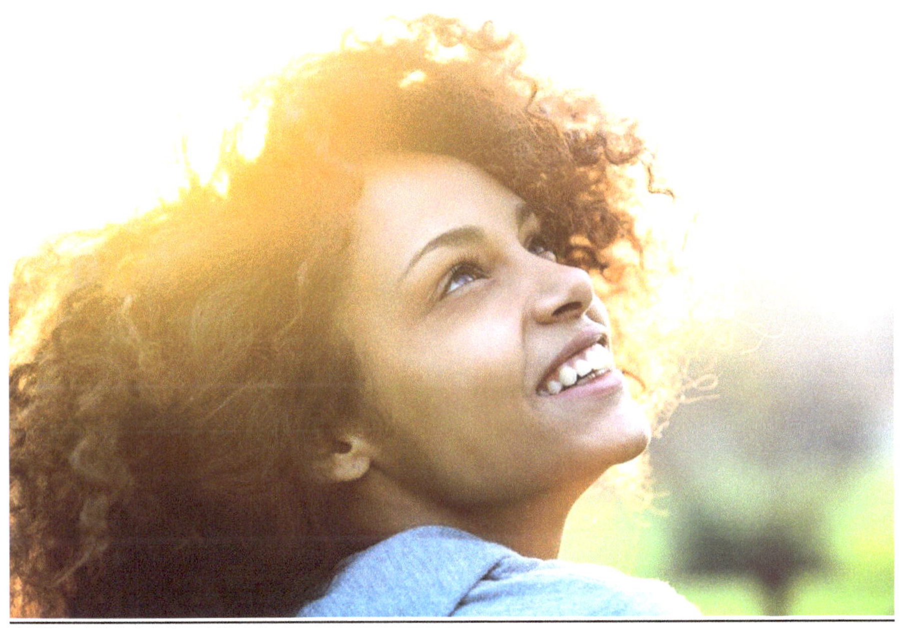

You don't need to be told that French women have a unique approach to staying young, healthy and beautiful. You will agree with me that it is intriguing the fact that despite how minimal the quantity of makeup and cosmetic they apply, they still appear to be perfect and their skin and hair looking glamorous, no wonder every girl wants to look flawless like the French women. It is hard not to say that every young girl wants to travel to France to acquire the first-hand lesson on how this magic is done and made to look so effortlessly. The good news is that you don't have to go to France now to know how it is done, here I am going to show you all the tips and tricks that will make you look radiant as revealed by our set of trusted French celebrity makeup artists

Preferred cosmetics

France houses quite a sizeable cosmetic industry, and you will pretty much find cream for almost everything, almost every French woman have a bottle of mineral water spray to help them moisturize the skin and keep her ever radiant.

As opposed to some of the general practice and believe, French women don't depend on make-ups and cosmetics for a total facial makeover, they will rather enhance their skin and face, and this begins with the use of healthy skin care routines, cosmetics, and products. Here are some of the most important brands and cosmetics that guarantee you the look of a French princess.

Astringent masks

An astringent cream mask, which contains high contents of active material/substances with an astringent effect.

This an efficient beautifying cream helps magnify and tone the skin. It also helps reduce pores and it is highly recommended for people with an oily and problematic skin, leaving your skin spotless, and all age group uses them. A gentle application of it for 15 to 20 minutes is all it takes after which you can wash it off with water or a tonic cleanser.

Retinol serum

This is lightweight and quickly absorbing serum with the effects of retinoid but which are now tolerant to sunlight. These are perfect moisturizers for the skin because they are made from extract and oils from tropical plants and ingredients rich in vitamins A, C and E. They are used as moisturizers and antioxidants for producing a smoothening and brightening effect to the skin. This cream will help reduce or possibly eliminate the formation of wrinkles and pores on your skin and reducing the pigmentation. They are suitable for all types of skin and can be applied to either the entire face or the infected part.

Enzymatic peeling

This is a very efficient emulsion made from a combination of active substances, compounds, and mixtures, which accelerates the dead removal cells and make for the regeneration of the skin. This cream is made for all ages and all skin types. The enzymes and acids they contain make it possible to remove keratinized skin. They are highly efficient in their moisturizing and complexion harmonizing. They should be used once in every five days and not be exposed to sunlight when they have been applied to the skin

When it comes to cream and oil brands highly recognized and preferred by the French women, RYOR is no sludge, This soft cream containing avocado, squalene and jojoba oils protects the skin against the effect of free radicals and its E vitamins and UV filter help reduce the effect of solar radiation on the skin. They are perfect for all skin types and age group and the best of it all, the product doesn't have any additives, no mineral oil or any synthetic perfume.

The French Woman lifestyle keeping them from others

To the French woman, a little bit of maquillage that the French women wear daily, the discrete foundation, mascara, and touch of eyeliner, a little bit of blush and gloss is all it takes to get you going for the day. The fascinating thing is the way the French woman blend and adapts their look to match the occasion even if it is grocery shopping. And this my friend, is what set a tone of difference between the French women and their counterparts from all over the world

Secrets on how to live and stay young

The secrets of the French are multifaceted. One of the important principles is that prevention is much more effective than the subsequent treatment. Therefore, they regularly and tirelessly take care of their face and body: daily masks, massage, and lymphatic drainage for the prevention of cellulite, thorough cleansing of the face from makeup before bed.

Maintain a French diet

Following a French diet can be key to living healthy; you need not be told that you are what you eat. The French understand this, and they ensure they diet on meals that keep their body and soul together. A demonstration of this good diet habit can be seen in a Mediterranean-style diet, which primarily consists of fish, olive, fresh vegetables, whole grains, nuts, legume and so on.

Pay attention to your water

The French women understand that water from natural sources contains likes of calcium, sodium magnesium, potassium and all that is required for healthy living, so they opt for water of natural sources such as celestins and hepar. They drink 6-8 glasses of water per day.

Give attention to your skin

The French women understand the importance of taking due and proper care of the skin. They understand that not only does it does it spell well for the general well-being of the body but it also makes for a glamorous look, and that is why they never leave for a vacation or any travel without prepping the skin for the journey.

Face massage

In the evening after a long working day, the best way to relax and your skin is to massage. It helps to not only relieve tension, but also to make the skin more elastic, relieve swelling, and with regular procedures even allows you to change the contour of the face. Everyone can have their technique of massage, but most importantly, what is worth remembering is the change of intense pressure on lighter massage movements.

Do not leave the red wine out

French wine is considered one of the best in the world. Many women drink it to keep the skin healthy and beautiful. One glass of a fragrant drink a day is the main secret of the youth of charming Madame and Mademoiselle. But not a drop more, because the effect can be directly opposite

French women love to pamper themselves.

Although they do not abuse cosmetics, great pleasure will be given to them to soak in the bath with fragrant oils, a pleasant smell of soap or body lotion, and a delicious smell of perfume.

Accept your imperfection

The French women accept their shortcomings and they have learned to manage and lay more emphasis on the unique aspect of their beauty instead of focusing on what they are not or trying to modify that part of the body, they have a problem.

Therefore, now you are convinced that the secrets of the beauty of French women are available to every woman. You just need a great desire and diligence!

Be your
own kind
of beautiful
♡

Copyright © 2018 by Sofi Bell.

All rights Reserved. No part of this publication or the information in it may be quoted from or reproduced in any form by means such as printing, scanning, photocopying or otherwise without prior written permission of the copyright holder.

Disclaimer and Terms of Use: Effort has been made to ensure that the information in this book is accurate and complete, however, the author and the publisher do not warrant the accuracy of the information, text and graphics contained within the book due to the rapidly changing nature of science, research, known and unknown facts and internet. The Author and the publisher do not hold any responsibility for errors, omissions or contrary interpretation of the subject matter herein. This book is presented solely for motivational and informational purposes only.